Keto Diet 2019 The Complete Keto Diet

Guide For Beginners Keto Diet

21-day meal plan step by step

Meal,breakfast,lunch, dinner and dessert

2 in 1

J.S. JOZEF

2

Copyright © 2019

Table of Contents

Introduction

The world we live in is one where we have access to junk and unhealthy foods without stress, while healthy foods are cloaked to look very distasteful. Gone are those days when you had to sacrifice good taste, all in the name of eating healthily.

Have you heard so much about ketogenic lifestyle to the extent that you are wondering if it is worth the hype? Journey with us, and we will show you why you need to join those that are benefitting from this healthy diet.

Chapter one

What is a Ketogenic Diet

For a lot of us that love to eat healthily, and lose weight, we must have heard of Ketogenic lifestyle. Day in, day out, you may wonder what ketogenic lifestyle is all about. You are in luck, as we will analyze every aspect.

One can say that the keto diet is one that integrates adequate protein and high fat, with very little carbs, and we won't be wrong.

The emphasis on the ketogenic diet is to reduce or strip your food of carbs while adding a high amount of fats to it.

When the ketogenic diet began, its creators weren't interested in using it to lose weight initially but had something in mind for it.

Ketogenic lifestyle was created to help treat epilepsy in kids. When a person consumes more and more of fats, the carbs that were once occupying a large part of the body mass is burnt. It gets to the stage, where the body no longer has carbs or glucose to burn. Hence it opts for the stored fat. The body focuses on the fat, burning it to act as a source of energy.

Usually, when a person is not subscribing to the ketogenic lifestyle, the person may tend to consume foods that are high in carbs. These carbs are turned to glucose. The glucose is moved around the body system, and it is used as fuel. The brain needs fuel to function.

When a person embraces a ketogenic lifestyle, his or her diet has little or no carbs. The body is forced to use the stored up fat as fuel.

The liver is forced to turn the fats, at this moment, to ketones and fatty acids. The ketones act as an energy source or fuel for the brain.

These ketones are transported to the brain, and they take the place of glucose. This means that the brain can depend on ketones, the same way it depends on glucose as a fuel source.

Once the ketone level in the body is high, the body is said to be in a state of ketosis. At this state, you will notice that a person is reducing in weight. For those kids suffering from epilepsy, when they are in a state of ketosis, there is a reduced level of seizures.

Research has shown that about half of those living with epilepsy that used this diet form had the rate of their seizures reduced by about half. The results didn't even change when they quit the diet. The Atkins diet offered them similar effect too. Know a child or young person that has epilepsy? The ketogenic diet can help.

For those that were suffering from pediatric epilepsy, the normal diet that was prescribed to them had the right amount of protein to help the child grow, while still given the right amount of calories to be at the right height and weight for their age.

The first type of therapeutic keto meal was designed to treat epilepsy in the early 1920s. It was used a lot to treat the ailment, but its usage reduced when drugs like anticonvulsant medications were made.

Keto diet is usually created to have high fat and low carbs. What is done is that there is an exclusion of foods that are high in carbs like starchy veggies, fruits, pasta, bread, sugar, as well as butter.

What "keto" means

The word, 'keto' in the keto diet means that the body will be forced to make use of ketones, which are tiny fuel molecules. This acts as another fuel for the human body, and takes the place of glucose when it is not in the right amount.

These energy molecules called, 'ketones' are made only when you eat little carbs. This means that if you consume a high amount if carbs, ketones can't be produced.

While the fat in the food acts as the energy source, the excess protein is turned into blood sugar.

The liver is the organ that is used in producing ketones from fat. Those tiny molecules produced are then transported around the body, including the brain.

The brain is one organ that is always hungry. Hence it needs a lot of energy daily. It is unable to run on fats but is capable of working well on glucose or ketones.

Once your body realizes that you are on a ketogenic diet, it has no other choice but to opt for fat, as it is a source of fuel. Immediately the insulin level plunges because the consumption of carbs has reduced, burning of fat increases.

At this stage, it is a lot easier if your fat stores are accessed, and burnt off quite easily.

This is awesome if you have decided to shed weight, as it can help you lose the excess weight. It is also great if you want to curtail your hunger, and still, have the necessary supply of energy.

A lot of persons who subscribe to the ketogenic lifestyle can testify that they are always focused and alert.

Immediately the body has started churning out ketones; it belongs to a stage christened, 'ketosis.' A lot of persons get into this stage quickly by fasting, but it's unable to fast forever. Fasting comes with a lot of issues that may affect your health.

This is where the ketogenic diet comes into play. You can continue the ketogenic lifestyle for a long while, enter the state of ketosis, and stay there. The ketogenic diet will give you what you wish- losing weight.

Possible therapeutic uses of the ketogenic diet
The ketogenic diet has been linked to the treatment of quite several neurological disorders like Parkinson's disease, Alzheimer's disease, brain cancer, pain, autism, amyotrophic lateral sclerosis, and even sleep disorders.

Epilepsy

Like earlier said, epilepsy is ranked as one of the commonest neurological disorders, following the ailment, stroke. It is said to be affecting millions of persons all over the world. One obvious symptom of epilepsy is unprovoked and regular seizures.

Seizures usually happen when a person has seizures, and this could affect the functioning of the brain. When seizures occur, the senses, muscles, or even consciousness may be affected. In the worst cases, three of them are affected.

Sometimes, the seizure can be restricted to a part of the brain, and in this case, it is called focal. Sometimes, it may spread around the entire brain, and in this case, it is generalized. Once a person has a generalized seizure, he or she may lose consciousness.

Causes of Epilepsy

The neurological condition can happen because of some reasons.

A lot of them started in one's childhood.

When one says that the case of epilepsy is refractory, it means that it has refused to be treated. This is a case when you have tried out about three or so anticonvulsant drugs, and they have all seemed to fail.

Statistics show that over sixty percent of the patients are known to get the control that they wish over their epilepsy using the first drug prescribed to them. Thirty percent of those with epilepsy do not get the necessary control using drugs.

When they realize that the drugs have failed, other options can be used. Some opt for the ketogenic diet, vagus nerve stimulation, as well as epilepsy surgery.

History of Ketogenic Diet

Ketogenic Diet came into limelight as a means of treating epilepsy. A lot of persons in the past made use of fasting to treat epilepsy, and it came with a lot of negative effects. When these were realized, a new method- a ketogenic lifestyle was created. It was meant to recreate the same success that fasting had created as a form of treating epilepsy.

It was very popular when it was created down to the 1930s, but its popularity waned when new anticonvulsant medications were created.

A lot of those that have epilepsy are capable of controlling their seizures by the use of medications.

For those that haven't been able to get the needed control, other methods are used.

Chapter Two
The 7-Day Keto Meal Plan

It has been noted that the ketogenic diet may be used by a lot of persons today to shed weight, it still has more uses. For those that want to embrace the ketogenic lifestyle, they may face challenges of how to create their first seven days meal plan. They are not to be planned, as being a first-timer in a tradition can do that.

Like earlier said, the ketogenic diet must have high fat, low carbs, and moderate protein. If it doesn't have any of the following, then it is not a ketogenic diet. If for any reason, you consume a food that is high in carbs, you may no longer be in the state of ketosis.

Let's say that the food you consume daily is 1,600 calories; you should eat about 100 grams of protein. It shouldn't be more than that, but it can be less.

You should consume about twenty-five grams of carbs. The number of carbs you consume shouldn't be more than that, but it can be less, while the fat you consume should be about 125 grams.

You can decide to mix any meal that you see on different days. They mustn't religiously follow.

All in all, it is expected that the daily macros be adjusted to meet your body needs.

You are expected to eat one serving for the recipes penned down, except when you are told otherwise.

DAY 1 DIETS

For Breakfast, eat

Keto Brunch Spread. The fat should be about 38g. Protein should be about 17g. Carbs should be about 3g, while calories should be about 426.

For lunch, eat Crispy Skin Salmon with Pesto Cauliflower Rice.

Fat should be about 51g. Protein should be about 24g. Carbs about 10g. Calories about 647.

For dinner, eat Superfood Meatballs and Keto Creamed Spinach.

The fats should be about 36g. Protein about 36g, and carbs about 7g. The calories should be about 485.

The total amount of macros that should be contained for the day are:

For fat, it should be 125g.

For protein, it should be 87g.

For carbs, it should be 20g.

The total amount of calories should be 1558.

DAY 2 MEALS

For breakfast, you should eat Chocolate Pancakes with Blueberry Butter.

The fats should be about 50g.

The protein should be about 27g.

Carbs should be about 11.5g

The calories should be about 611.

For lunch, eat Turkey Sausage Frittata and four slices bacon.

They should be fried in a tablespoon of butter, and you can use a cup of coffee while eating them.

The fats should be about 50g.

The protein should be about 25g.

The carbs should be about 5.5g, while total calories are 572.

For dinner, try out Lemon Herb Low Carb Keto Meatloaf.

The fats should be about 29g.

The protein should be about 33g.

The fats should be about 2g, while calories are about 344.

For the entire day, you should have total macros of:

Fats should be 129g

Protein should be 85g

Carbs should be 19g

Calories should be 1,527.

DAY 3 MEALS

For Breakfast, you should consider eating Bacon, Egg & Cheese Breakfast Casserole.

The fat in it should be 38g.

The protein in it should be 43g.

The carbs in it should be 4g, while the number of calories in it should be 437.

For Lunch, you can try out White Turkey Chili. It should be cooked with a tablespoon of olive oil, and two cups of mixed leafy greens.

The number of fats should be 44.5g.

Protein should be 28.8g.

Fats should be 5.5g, while calories are 568.

For dinner, try out Portobello Bun Cheeseburger with Celeriac. Ensure that everything there has been oven fried, and spice it with Homemade Keto Mayo.

The amount of fat there should be 40g.

Protein should be 31g, while carbs should be 13g. The calories are 539.

The entire macros for the day's consumption should be:

122.5 grams for fat consumption,

102.8 grams for protein consumption, 20.5 grams for carbs consumption, and 1,544 total calories consumed.

DAY 4 MEALS

For breakfast, you can decide to go for Keto Power Breakfast Bowl.

The number of fats should be 27g.

Protein should be 10.5g.

Carbs should be 7g, and calories should be 305.

For lunch, you can try out the Crispy Cheesy Chicken Salad.

For fat, it should contain 36.5g.

For protein should be 55g.

For carbs, it should be 8g.

As for calories, the total should be 575.

For dinner, you should try out Grilled ribeye steak- Four ounces, Mixed leafy greens- Two cups, Grass fed butter- Two tablespoons, and Avocado oil- A tablespoon.

For fat, it should have 62g.

For protein, it should be 20g.

For carbs, it should be a gram, and as for calories, the total should be about 636.

For Dessert, try out MCT Fat Bomb.

The fats should be 8g.

Protein should be 1g.

Carbs should be 2g.

Total calories should be 81.

For the entire day, the macros should be 133.5 grams for fat. As for protein and the total calories, they should be 86.5g and 1597 respectively.

DAY 5 MEALS

For breakfast, try out Avocado Breakfast Bowl.

The fat should be about 40g.

Protein should be about 25g.

Carbs should be about 3g.

The total calories should be about 500.

For lunch, try out the Roasted Chicken Stacks.

The fat should be 25g.

The protein should be 34g.

The carbs should be 5.5g.

Calories should be 369.

For dinner, try out the Cheesy Broccoli Meatza

For fat, it should be 24g.

For protein, it should be 32g.

For carbs, it should be 7g.

For calories, it should be 375.

For dessert, try out Two Macadamia Nut Fat Bombs.

Fats should be 34g.

Protein should be 2g.

Carbs should be 4g, while calories are 200.

For the entire day, the macros should be 123 grams for fat.

For protein, it should be 93 grams.

For carbs, it should be 19.5 grams, and calories are 1,444.

DAY 6 MEALS

For breakfast, try out Acai Almond Butter Smoothie.

For fat, it should be 40g.

For protein, it should be 15g.

For carb, it should be 6g, and calories should be 345.

For lunch, try out Keto Beef Bulgogi.

For fat, it should be 18g.

For protein, it should be 25g.

For carbs, it should be 3g, while the total amount of calories are 242.

For a snack, try out one ounce of almonds, and one hard-boiled egg.

For fat, it should be 19g.

For protein, it should be 12g.

For carbs, it should be 3g. Calories are 241.

For dinner, try out Creamy Mushroom Chicken.

For fat, it should be 27g.

For protein, it should be 24g.

For carbs, it should 3g.

Total calories are 241.

For Dessert, try out the Keto Chocolate Mousse.

For fats, it should be 14g.

For protein, it should be 17.5g.

For carbs, it should be 6g.

The total calories are 248.

For the entire, the macros are meant to be 98 grams for fat,

93.5 grams for protein,

21 grams for carbs.

The total calories should be 1,410.

DAY 7 MEALS

For Breakfast, try out Keto Bulletproof Coffee.

The fat should be 31g.

The protein should be 1g.

The carb should be 0.5g, while total calories are 280.

For Lunch, try out Low Carb Crispy Keto "Fried" Chicken, then top it with a cup of steamed broccoli.

For fat, it is 37g.

For protein, it should be 33.5g.

For carbs, it should be 6.5g.

For calories, it should be 494.

For dinner, try out Low Carb Keto Lasagna.

For fats, it should be 21g.

For protein, it should be 32g.

For carbs, it should be 12g.

For the total calories, it should be 364.

For dessert, try out Collagen Mug Cake.

For fats, it should be 43.5g.

For protein, it should be 27g.

For carbs, it should be 4g.

Total calories should be 535.

The macros for the entire day are:

Fats should be 122.5g.

Protein should be 93.5g.

Carbs should be 23g.

The total calories are 1,673.

There is one thing that should be noted, you will rarely meet your daily macro goal, but you shouldn't be scared. What you should do as a rule is to ensure that your protein and carbs goals are met to an extent.

You can easily look at the numbers if you wish.

Since you now know how a ketogenic diet week should look like, planning the next week should be a lot easier.

Chapter three

Keto food preparation

Research-Backed Reasons to Meal Prep on Keto

A lot of persons have the wrong thought that only motivation can get them to lose weight, and when they realize that it is a fallacy, you see them adding more weight than when they decided to shed the weight.

Don't think it is only you that have gone through such. For years, I have heard people complain that they thought motivation could get them through. The basic truth remains that motivation isn't everything.

You can't be motivated every blessed minute in the day, and that's the basic truth.

If you want to succeed on this journey, there has to be some plan. You don't have to rely on motivation to get the job done solely. A study that was done by the British Journal of Health Psychology stated that about ninety percent of those that participated in an exercise that was scheduled was known to work weekly, even if it was just once while those that didn't have any exercise scheduled had problems exercising, even if it was once a week.

If after this, you still need reasons you need to get up and start the meal prep immediately, below are awesome reasons:

#1: MEAL PREP CONQUERS DECISION FATIGUE

Do you that decision fatigue is a real thing? How? You may ask. Have you ever wondered why the likes of Mark Zuckerberg, Obama, and even Steve Jobs, while alive, wear the same clothes daily? The stress that comes with picking out cloth is exhausting. Hence they just buy similar clothes. This stops them from having to decide on what they should have on.

Humans are known to have restricted willpower, and if they are made to make decisions regularly, they get bored of it. The next decision they make becomes a chore, and before you know it they start asking if they even made the right decision. What would have happened if they had opted for the alternative?

Researchers decided to see what made prisoners become paroled, and it was noticed that there was a trend. After looking at more than a thousand decisions, it was noticed that prisoners were released parole based on a trend. Based on the report published by the New York Times, those prisoners that came before the judge in the morning were able to receive paroles a lot. About 70% was given parole. While those prisoners that came later on in the day had to battle with about ten percent or even less, this means that paroles were given to prisoners, not because of their crimes, but when they arrived.

When we look at it, we can see that the number of decisions that the judge had made earlier on in the day had forced him to see other decisions that he was to make as unappealing. This is basic psychology.

Have you ever gone to an office in the afternoon for something, and you saw them all angry, and tired of you immediately you entered there. Have you also gone to that office another day in the morning, and realized that they were happy to meet you?

Why is this so? No one likes to make decisions after making a string of decisions.

The same way the judge's willpower was reduced when he continuously made decisions is the same way you get tired of making decisions after a while.

The reason some persons quit keto is not that it's not effective, but the fact that they have to make choices when it comes to their food becomes tiring.

How can they save themselves the stress? The answer is very simple. You can create a meal plan, and you are good to go.

Your meal plan reduces the number of choices that need to be made. This makes your willpower to remain intact. If you want to adopt a ketogenic lifestyle, you need a meal plan.

2. Meal Prep Allows You Save Both Money and Time

Do you know that a typical person spends a lot of time and money making decisions? Let's say you refused to make a meal plan; you won't know what you want to eat. Hence you may end up spending a lot more money and time than necessary. Smart persons try to make a meal plan for weeks at a stretch, as it allows them to budget. If you know that you will be eating this and this, you can easily buy them in bulk and store. For those foods that can be cooked and stored in the refrigerator. You can always bring them out and microwave when you want to eat.

This allows you to save time that would have been wasted in shopping daily, cooking every time or looking for what meal to eat.

Planning your meal stops you from wasting food. This could help you save your money, but it can do much more.

For those that believe in saving the environment, food wastage is something that we should try and avoid.

When you plan, you save yourself this stress.

Planning your meals allows you to know what you intend to buy, and make you stick to those things that are important. It allows you to know how much you should spend for your groceries weekly.

3. Preparing for meals help you to reach the state of ketosis.

One thing that a lot of persons face is calculating their macros. It can be annoying to calculate them. Meal prep can help.

When you have a meal plan, it is quite easy for you to know what your macro goals are, and stick to them. You don't just make decisions out of nowhere that could affect your macro goals.

Simple Steps for Easy Keto Meal Prep
Everyone doesn't have to follow the same path while making their meal preps. This is to act as a guideline when deciding what to eat.

Start by deciding what you intend to eat.

You should start on the first day of the week. Write the day down, and think of what you should eat then. Write them down for breakfast down to dinner. Do it for the next six days.

Make up your mind on what you will eat every day for breakfast, lunch, and dinner. This should also include the desserts or snacks you may wish to consume.

You can put it in a calendar if you wish. On the other hand, you can have it broken down to every day that week.

Find out the calories of the foods you have chosen, and their composition. Remember that the fat content should be the highest, followed by protein and carbs.

Write out how many persons will munch on the food, and if you intend to have leftovers that can be consumed the day after, or if a new food will be consumed daily.

Ensure that the meal is kept simple by you eating the same food more than once in a week. This will allow you to save on the time that will be spent cooking, and you can dine on the leftovers. If you don't have the time or money to make mee foods every time, this can save you the stress. If, on the other hand, you have the time and money, you can make new delicacy every time without stress.

It is important that you pen down the recipes for the food that you will want to prepare. Don't forget to pin down the ingredients that will be used to prepare it. This will allow you to know what you need to prepare the food. You can easily source for the ingredients in bulk at the store and save yourself the stress.

Some persons don't mind doing everything in a day, and there are others that like to divide up the work.

A tip that can be used to your advantage is to choose those recipes that are easy to make and come bearing a few ingredients. You can opt for those recipes that have similar ingredients. Hence you can use them to make different foods.

You can decide to opt for recipes that use the same veggies or meats.

This allows the shopping list to be a lot shorter, and food can be cooked quickly.

In the end, you will be left with a shorter shopping list.

Create The List, Then Shop

Now that you have chosen the recipes you want and their ingredients, you can have your shopping list compiled. Have them broken down into groups, and you can begin the list with those that you see immediately you enter into the grocery shop.

Don't forget to pen down the amount of ingredient you want, and ensure that your shopping revolves around the list. Opt for the whole foods, and try to avoid packaged foods. A lot of packaged foods may claim to be keto friendly, but they are far from that.

One method that I have used for a long time to shop is to immediately walk towards the produce and butcher sections, without looking at the packaged foods. This prevents me from stocking up on packaged foods and ignoring fresh produce or meat.

Prepare Your Meals

A lot of persons feel that shopping is the difficult part of the process, while some others, feel that it is the stage of preparing the meals. For those that opt for the former, it is not surprising because a lot of persons hate the thoughts of leaving their home and heading to the store. The thought of pushing the trolley annoys them. To some others, it may be the fact that there are a lot of options available, and before you know it, they have stocked their trolleys with unnecessary things.

For those that feel that cooking is the problem. We won't blame them. Maybe, they don't have a flair for cooking or cooking seems scary for them. Whichever way, cooking shouldn't be scary, especially when you have the recipe in front of you.

Cooking is one tricky process, but once you get used to it, it becomes so simple that you can cook while you sleepwalk.

Below are some tips that should be considered:

Get out the recipe, and read it. Before you bring out anything or start doing anything, try and understand every process. This prevents you from being stuck at a place or making mistakes.

Let's say that in the recipe, it states that you should slow cook the chicken. This should be something that you do first before you think of chipping the veggies or having the cauliflower rice made. This ensures that time isn't wasted.

Take out every ingredient that you will need before you start cooking. Go to the pantry and bring them out. If they are in the fridge, do the same.

If the recipe needs the veggies to be chopped, or the meats to be pre-cooked, you should consider doing that. This allows you to use them when you want easily.

Immediately you are done preparing the meal; it is advisable to store them in different containers. This will allow the foods to stay for a while.

You can have every container labeled with a sticky note to allow you to remember what it contains. You should also pen what day the food is meant for, as well as when it was made, and even the macros.

Meal Prep Money Saving Tips

A lot of persons feel that eating healthily or subscribing to the ketogenic lifestyle. What of if we told you that this is a pure fallacy?

Keto lifestyle is a very affordable one if you know what to do, or what to seek for. If you want to save money, while you eat healthily, then these tips will help.

Opt for those recipes that have seasonal produce. The trick of shopping is buying mostly those things that are in season. Why is this so? When something is in season, it tends to be a lot cheaper, and available. During the season for a food item, you can purchase a large amount of it for little or nothing, but when out of season, the opposite is the case.

You will likely see a lot of them on sale. Go to the grocery store and purchase them. Ensure that you have where to store them to prevent them from going stale.

Head To The Farmer's Market. This is one place that you should frequent. Many grocery stores get their produce from farmers, and when you decide to cut the middlemen out, you can get fresh foods without paying a lot. You may think that there's no farmer's market near you, but I doubt that. All you need to do is ask, and you will find. When you get there, be friendly with those in the market, and you will get great deals on fresh foods, especially dairy products.

Stay off packaged foods

The truth remains that one can't stay off packaged food, but you can reduce the amount that you consume. Apart from the fact that packaged foods are far from healthy, they aren't cheap. You may say that they have been cleaned and bagged. Hence the are easier to use, but have you considered the hole that it is digging in your pocket.

They may seem convenient, but they aren't so affordable. You can get fresh food, and save yourself some money. Usually, when you compare how much you spend on processed foods and fresh ones, you will realize that the disparity is much.

Search around for coupons or discounts

Stores are known to churn out special offers, but you may not know of them. Some persons only find out when they search or head to the store.

You can visit the store's website to seek for those offers. To get a regular stream of such information, save yourself the trouble, and sign up for their email newsletters. It may seem like an inconvenience, but you won't know when you will get those deals.

Purchase in the large amount

This is a smart trick that buyers have used for a long time. When items are being purchased in bulk, discounts are given to the buyer. You can head to the farmer's market or grocery store and purchase the ingredients in bulk. Before you do this, it is important that you have where to store them. Don't go and buy those items that will end up spoiling because you don't have storage space.

Have your items grown

If you fall under those with green thumbs, you will enjoy growing your food. It will help you save money that would have been expended in a store. Forget about the money saved, do you know that it is healthier to consume home grown foods than the one bought in the store? A lot of store foods are genetically modified and have been stripped of part of their nutrients. Some are toxic to the body because of the chemicals that have been added to grow them.

If you have a yard, you should think of growing herbs and veggies there. You don't have to have a big yard before you can do it. There are currently a lot of space managing tips online that help those with tiny space grow their foods.

You can also make your food. Yes, you read that right. Instead of heading to the store to get the processed varieties, you can make things like

- Mayo,

- Bone broth,

- Ketchup,

- Salad dressings and sauces,

- Bacon,

- Mustard,

- Sauerkraut,

- Pesto,

- Ghee,

- Coconut flour,

- Almond milk and so on.

There are tips on how to make them online.

Chapter Four:

Keto breakfast recipes

We have discussed some life-saving tips that you can use to lead a healthy lifestyle without breaking the bank. Now, we will look at those healthy ketogenic breakfast recipes that you should consider.

A lot of persons believe that keto recipes have to stale to the tongue. Far from it, keto wants you to lead a healthy lifestyle, and it also wants you to eat delicious foods. You may have shied away from other healthy lifestyles because of how averse they were to the taste bud, but this is different.

Keto cereal

You can treat your taste buds to the good things of life, and treat your body to a healthy diet. All you have to do is try out the keto cereal, and you will be impressed.

What You Need

- Chopped Almonds- One c.

- Sesame seeds- Quarter c.

- Walnuts- One c.

- Unsweetened coconut flakes- One c.

- Chia seeds- Two tablespoons

- Flax seeds- Two tablespoons

- Ground clove- One and a half teaspoon

- Cinnamon- One and a half teaspoon

- Egg white- One

- Kosher salt- Half teaspoon

- Coconut oil- Quarter c

- Cooking spray

Directions

Start by having the oven preheated to 250. Get out your baking sheet, and line it with cooking spray.

Take out a big bowl, and toss in your coconut flakes, almonds, flax seeds, sesame seeds, walnuts, as well as chia seeds.

Whisk in your vanilla, cinnamon, salt, as well as cloves.

Whisk the egg white till it becomes foamy, then add it to the granola. Whisk in the coconut oil, and don't stop until they are coated well.

Put the mixture on the baking sheet, and ensure that it is well layered.

Allow it bake for about twenty-five minutes. Ensure that it is golden before you bring it out. Allow it cool well before you serve.

Best-Ever Cabbage Hash Browns

What You Need

- Kosher salt- Half teaspoon
- Eggs- Two
- Galic powder- Half teaspoon
- Pepper- to taste

- Vegetable oil- One tablespoon

- Yellow onion- Quarter

- Shredded cabbage- Two c.

Directions

Get out a big bowl and stir your garlic powder, eggs, and salt. Toss in the black pepper, before you add the onion and cabbage. Ensure you mix well, and don't stop.

Take out a big skillet, and put it on a stove with medium heat. Add your oil, and allow it heat for a while.

Have the mixture divided into four patties in that pan that you have decided to use? Make use of your spatula and have them flattened. Allow them to cook till they become tender and golden for over three minutes. You should then turn to the other side.

Keto pancakes

What You Need

- Almond flour- Half c

- Eggs- Four

- Cream cheese- Four ounces

- Lemon zest- One teaspoon.

- Butter

Directions

Take out a medium bowl, and stir in the eggs, cream cheese, lemon zest, and almond flour. Continue to stir till they become smooth.

Take out your nonstick skillet and place it on a stove with medium heat. Have a tbsp of butter melted on it, then add three tablespoons of the batter. Allow them to cook for about two minutes or till you notice that they have taken the golden hue.

Toss them to the other side, and allow them to cook for about two minutes again.

Put them in a plate, then continuously cook the rest of the batter.

You can top them with butter.

Keto smoothie

What You Need

- Strawberries- Two c.
- Raspberries- Two c
- Blackberries- Two c
- Baby spinach- One c
- Coconut milk- Two c
- Orange juice
- Unsweetened shaved coconut. This is to garnish. Hence it is optional.

Directions

Take out a blender and add all these ingredients. Leave the coconut out of the mixture. Blend them till you notice that they are smooth.

Take out your cups and fill. You can garnish them with coconut and raspberries.

Keto breakfast cup

What You Need

- Ground pork- Two lb
- Chopped thyme- One tablespoon
- Garlic- Two cloves
- Paprika- Half teaspoon
- Cumin- Half teaspoon

- Salt- One teaspoon

- Fresh spinach- Chopped.

- Two and a half c

- Black pepper- to taste

- Shredded cheddar- One c

- Eggs- Twelve

- Chopped chives- A tablespoon

Directions

Start by preheating the oven until it reaches a temperature of 200. Take out a big bowl, and add your cumin, paprika, garlic, thyme, ground pork, as well as salt. Toss in the pepper.

Take out a bit of the pork and place them on every muffin tin. Have every side pressed up to form a cup. Have the cheese and spinach divided up well among the cups?

Get an egg, and crack it on every cup. Add pepper and salt to taste. Do the same for the remaining eggs.

Leave them in the oven, and allow them to bake well. This should take over twenty-five minutes. Add your chives, then serve.

Keto blueberry muffin

What You Need

- Almond flour- Two and a half c.
- Sugar- One-third c. Keto friendly

- Baking powder- One and a half teaspoons

- Salt- Half teaspoon

- Baking soda- Half teaspoon

- Melted butter- One this c.

- Almond milk- One third c

- Eggs- Three

- Vanilla extract- A teaspoon

- Blueberries- One teaspoon

- Lemon zest- Half

- Blueberries- Two-third c.

Directions

Have your oven preheated to 150. Take out your muffin pan, and line it with cupcake liners.

Take out a big bowl, and toss in your Swerve, almond flour, salt, baking soda, baking powder.

Toss in your eggs, almond milk, butter, and vanilla. Don't stop until they are well mixed

Take out the lemon zest and blueberries and fold till well distributed.

Take out similar amounts of the batter in the cupcake liner, and put in the oven. Allow it bake for about twenty-three minutes. To be sure that they are ready, you can use a toothpick and insert it in the muffin. If it comes out clean, then it is ready.

Allow them to cool well before you serve.

Chapter Five

Keto Lunch Recipes

Loaded cauliflower bake

What You Need

- Cauliflower head- One. Cut to form florets

- Butter- Two tablespoons

- Heavy cream- One cup

- Cream cheese- Two ounces

- Sharp cheddar- One and quarter cup

- Pepper and salt

- Bacon- Six slices

- Green onions- Quarter cup

Directions

Start by preheating the oven until it reaches a high temperature of 150.

Take out a big pot and boil water. When it is boiling, put the cauliflower florets there for two minutes. After then, have the cauliflower drained.

Take out a medium pot, and melt the cream cheese, heavy cream, and butter. Stir in the pepper salt and cheddar cheese. Don't stop till they are well combined.

Take out your baking dish, and toss in the cheese sauce, cauliflower florets, then add every crumbled bacon and green onions, but save one tablespoon of each somewhere else. Stir the mixture together.

Add the extra crumbled bacon, cheddar cheese and green onions to them.

Allow them to bake till the cheese has become golden and bubbly. The cauliflower must be soft before you bring it out. This should take about thirty minutes.

Turkey Chili

What You Need

- Organic ground turkey- One lb

- Cauliflower- Two cups

- Coconut oil- Two tablespoons

- Vidalia onion- Half

- Garlic- Two cloves

- Coconut milk- Two cups

- Mustard- A tablespoon

- Salt- One teaspoon

Directions

Start by heating the coconut oil in a big pot.

While it heats, cut the garlic and onion, then put them in the hot oil.

Continue to stir them for about two minutes before you put the ground turkey.

Have the mixture broken up using the spatula. Dong stop stirring till you see that it is crumbled.

Put the seasoning mix, as well as the riced cauliflower. Don't forget to stir well.

When you notice that the meat is now browned, put the coconut milk, and allow it to simmer for about eight minutes. Don't forget to stir.

Once it gets to this point, you can then serve. Add the shredded cheese to give it the thick sauce feel.

BBQ pulled beef Sando

Who said you have to eat bland foods all in the name of leading a ketogenic lifestyle? No one. Bask in the good things of life, and tasty foods with the BBQ pulled beef Sando.

What You Need

- Boneless Chuck Roast- Three lbs
- Pink Himalayan Salt- Two teaspoons
- Garlic powder- Two teaspoons
- Black pepper- One teaspoon
- Onion powder- One teaspoon
- Smoked paprika- One tablespoon
- Tomato paste- Two tablespoons
- Apple cider vinegar- Quarter cup
- Coconut aminos- Two tablespoons

- Bone broth- Half cup

- Butter- Quarter cup

Directions

Have the fat trimmed off the beef, before you cut them up into two big pieces.

Take out a small bowl, then toss in the ingredients like black pepper, onion, salt, paprika, and garlic. Leave the beef to cook in a slow cooker.

Take out another bowl, and have the butter melted. Don't forget to add the vinegar, tomato paste, as well as coconut aminos. Pour the mixture on the beef.

Allow it to cook for about ten hours, but it should be on low. When it is ready, take out the beef, and leave the slow cooker at a high temperature. This will allow it thicken. You can then have the beef shredded before you add it to the slow cooker. Put the sauce, and voilà, you are good to go.

You can then serve.

Chapter Six

Keto dinner recipes

Want to dine with your family healthily, yet satisfy your taste buds? Try out the following keto dinner recipes. They are affordable and easy to make.

Bell pepper eggs

What You Need

- Bell pepper- One

- Eggs- Six

- Kosher salt

- Black peppers

- Chopped chives- Two tablespoons

- Chopped parsley- Two tablespoons

Directions

Take out a skillet, and place it on a stove with medium heat. Ensure that you grease it well with cooking spray.

Take out the bell pepper ring and put in the skillet. Allow it sauté for about two minutes. Ensure that the ring is flipped before you crack the egg there in the middle.

Put your pepper and salt to season it, then allow it to cook for about three minutes, till you notice that egg has been cooked.

Do the same thing with the remaining eggs, and don't forget to have them garnished with parsley and chives.

Bunless bacon, egg, and cheese

What You Need

- Eggs- Twp

- Water- Two tablespoons

- Avocado- Half

- Cooked bacon- Two slices

- Cheddar cheese- Quarter C.

Directions

Take out a medium pan, and put two mason jar lids there. Ensure that you have removed the centers.

Using cooking spray, spray the pan, and put it on a stove with medium heat.

Bring the eggs, and have them cracked in the middle of the lids. Try and whisk it lightly using a fork to remove the yolk.

Around the lids, pour water and have the pan covered. Allow them to cook for a while till you notice that the whites have been cooked.

Take out the lid, and add the cheddar on the eggs. Allow them to cook until they become a bit melty. This can take about a minute.

Have the egg bun inverted on a plate without the cheese. Have it topped with cooked Bacon, as well as mashed avocado.

Top it using the cheesy egg bun, while the cheese faces side-down. You can munch on them with a fork and knife.

Cloud eggs

What You Need

- Eggs- Eight
- Parmesan- One c

- Deli ham- Half Lb

- Black pepper

- Kosher salt

- Chopped chives

Directions

Start by preheating the oven until it gets to 250.

Have the baking sheet greased with cooking spray.

Get the yolks and egg whites separated. Put the egg whites in a big bowl, and yolk in the small bowl. Use a hand mixer to whisk the egg whites for about three minutes or till you notice that stiff peaks have formed.

Add in the ham and Parmesan, then season with a bit of pepper and salt.

Take out about eight mounds of the egg whites into the baking sheet, and indent the centers to create nests. Allow them to bake for three minutes till you notice that they are golden.

Before you serve, garnish them with chives.

Cookie dough keto fat bomb

What You Need

- Butter- Eight tablespoons
- Keto friendly sweetener like Swerve- One-third c.

- Vanilla extract- Half teaspoon

- Kosher salt- Half teaspoon

- Almond flour- Two c

- Chocolate chips- Two third c

Directions

Take out a big bowl, and put the butter there. Beat it with a hand mixer till you notice that it is fluffy and light. Toss in the salt, vanilla, and sugar. Continue to beat till they combine well.

Gently whisk in the almond flour till you can't see any dry spot again. Add the chocolate chips.

Use a plastic wrap to cover the bowl, and leave it in the refrigerator for about twenty minutes to become quite firm.

Make use of a tiny cookie scoop to scoop the dough till it forms tiny balls. Leave it in the fridge, and it can stay for up to a week. If you want it to stay up to a month, leave in the freezer.

Bacon avocado bomb

What You Need

- Avocado- Two

- Bacon- Eight

- Cheddar- One third c

Directions

Start by heating the broiler. Take out your baking sheet, and have it lined with foil.

Have the avocado sliced into half, then take out the pits. Remove the skin from every avocado.

Ensures that the halves are filled with cheese, then put the other halves of the avocado. Have every avocado wrapped with bacon- four slices.

Put the avocado now wrapped in bacon in the baking sheet, and allow it broil till you notice that the bacon is now crispy. This should take about five minutes.

Gently, turn the avocado with tongs, and allow them to cook till crispy. This should take an extra five minutes.

Plain Cloud Bread

What You Need

- Three eggs
- Cream of tartar- Quarter teaspoon
- Kosher salt- A pinch
- Cream cheese- Two ounces

Directions

Start by preheating the oven to a high temperature of 200. Have your baking sheet lined with the parchment paper.

Take out two bowls, and separate the yolks from the egg whites. Put the salt and cream of tartar to the egg whites. Use a hand mixer to whisk well till you notice the stiff peaks. This should take about three minutes.

Toss in the cream cheese to egg yolks. Take out your hand mixer and whisk the cream cheese with the mix yolks till you notice that they are well combined. Gradually pour the egg yolk mixture to the egg whites.

Have the mixture divided into six mounds on the baking sheet. Ensure that they have been spaced about four inches away. Continue to bake for thirty minutes till you notice that they are golden.

Have each bread piece sprinkled with cheese. Leave it in the oven to bake for about two minutes, till the cheese melts.

Allow it cool before you serve.

Pizza Cloud Bread

What You Need

- Italian seasoning- One tablespoon
- Shredded mozzarella- Two tablespoons

- Parmesan- Two tablespoons

- Tomato paste- Two teaspoons

Directions

Break the egg, and put a tbsp of Italian seasoning, tomato paste, shredded mozzarella into the egg yolk mixture

Have the mixture divided into six mounds on the baking sheet. Ensure that they have been spaced about four inches away. Continue to bake for thirty minutes till you notice that they are golden.

Have each bread piece sprinkled with cheese. Leave it in the oven to bake for about two minutes, till the cheese melts.

Allow it cool before you serve.

Bagel Cloud Bread

What You Need

- Kosher salt- One-eight teaspoon

- Poppy seeds- One teaspoon

- Sesame seeds- One teaspoon

- Dried garlic- One teaspoon

- Dried onion- One teaspoon. Minced

Directions

Break the egg, and put it in a bowl. Add the poppy seeds, kosher salt, sesame seed, dried onion, and dried garlic to the mixture.

Have the mixture divided into six mounds on the baking sheet. Ensure that they have been spaced about four inches away. Continue to bake for thirty minutes till you notice that they are golden.

Have each bread piece sprinkled with cheese. Leave it in the oven to bake for about two minutes, till the cheese melts.

Allow it cool before you serve.

Ranch Cloud Bread

- Ranch seasoning powder- One and a half teaspoons
- Eggs

Directions

Break the egg in a big bowl, and add the ranch seasoning powder into the egg yolk mixture.

Have the mixture divided into six mounds on the baking sheet. Ensure that they have been spaced about four inches away. Continue to bake for thirty minutes till you notice that they are golden.

Have each bread piece sprinkled with cheese. Leave it in the oven to bake for about two minutes, till the cheese melts.

Allow it cool before you serve.

Chapter Seven

Keto Dessert Recipes

Keto diets also come in the form of desserts. This means that you can enjoy your dessert recipe without stress.

Keto avocado brownies

What You Need

- Eggs- Four

- Avocados- Two

- Butter- Half c. Melted

- Peanut butter- Six tablespoons- Six

- Baking soda- Two teaspoons

- Coconut sugar- Two- third c.

- Vanilla extract- Two teaspoons

- Cocoa powder- Two teaspoons

- Salt- Half teaspoon

Directions

Start by preheating the oven to a high temperature of 250. Get out your pan out, and have it lined with parchment paper. Take out your blender and toss in every ingredient, then blend till you notice that it is smooth.

Put the batter in the baking pan, and make use of a spatula to smoothen it.

Leave in the oven till you notice that the brownies are now soft, but they shouldn't be wet. This usually takes about twenty-five minutes. Before you serve, allow them to cool.

Chocolate mousse

What You Need

- Avocados- Two

- Heavy dream- Three-quarter c.

- Chocolate chips- Half c. Must be keto friendly.

- Honey- Quarter c

- Cocoa powder- Three tablespoons. Unsweetened.

- Honey- Quarter c.

- Kosher salt- Half teaspoon

Directions

Take out your blender and toss in every ingredient. Don't put the chocolate yet.

Blend them, toss in the chocolate, then blend again.

Pour it in your glasses, and allow it to sit in the refrigerator for a while before you serve.

Keto frosty

What You Need

- Whipping cream- One and a half c.

- Cocoa powder- Two tablespoons

- Sugar sweetener- Three tablespoons. Keto friendly

- Kosher salt- A pinch

- Vanilla extract- A teaspoon

Directions

Take out a big bowl, and toss in your salt, vanilla, sweetener, cocoa, and cream. Use a hand mixer and beat it till you notice stiff peaks forming. Take out your Ziploc bag, and pour the mixture in. Allow it freeze for thirty minutes.

Snip a part of the bag out, and put in the serving dishes.

Magic keto cookies

What You Need

- Coconut oil- Quarter c

- Butter- Four tablespoons. Softened

- Swerve sweetener- Two tablespoons

- Egg yolks- Four

- Coconut flakes- One c

- Dark chocolate chips- One c

- Coconut flakes- One c

- Chopped Walnuts- Three third c.

Directions

Start by preheating the oven until it reaches a high temperature of 250.

Take out a baking sheet, and have it lined with parchment paper.

Take out a big bowl, and whisk in egg yolks, sweetener, butter, and coconut oil. Add your walnuts, coconut and chocolate chips.

Put the batter into the baking sheet, and leave in the oven. Allow it to bake for about fifteen minutes or till it becomes golden.

Peanut butter cookies

What You Need

- Unsweetened Peanut- One and a half c

- Coconut flour- One c.

- Coconut sugar- Quarter c.

- Vanilla extract- One teaspoon

- Kosher salt- A pinch

- Chocolate chips- Two c.

- Coconut oil- A tablespoon

Directions

Take out a medium bowl, and toss in the salt, vanilla, coconut sugar, coconut flour, and peanut butter.

Take out your baking sheet and line with parchment paper. Make use of a tiny cookie scoop, and form the mixture to rounds before you press them down on the baking sheet. This will flatten them. Allow them to freeze for about one hour, or till you notice that it is firm.

Take out a medium bowl, and toss in the coconut oil and melted chocolate.

Making use of a fork, dip the rounded peanut butter in the chocolate till you notice that it has been properly coated. Take it back to the baking sheet.

Pour more peanut butter on them, and allow them to freeze till you notice that they are set. This usually takes ten minutes.

You can then serve cold. Allow them to stay in the freezer.

Chocolate mug cake

What You Need

- Butter- Two tablespoons
- Egg- One
- Cocoa powder- Two tablespoons
- Almond flour- Quarter c
- Chocolate chips- Two tablespoons. Keto friendly

- Baking powder- Half teaspoon

- Keto friendly sweetener- One teaspoon

- Kosher salt- A pinch

- Whipped cream- Quarter c

Directions

Take out a safe microwave mug and coat it with butter. Allow it to stay in a microwave for thirty seconds to melt. Put the other ingredients, and not the whipped cream. Continue to stir till you notice that they are fully mixed.

Allow it to cook for about a minute, till the cake is now set, but still having the fudgy feel.

Garnish with whipped cream.

You can then serve.

Keto ice cream

What You Need

- Coconut milk- Two. Fifteen ounces

- Heavy cream- Two c

- Sweetener- Keto friendly. Quarter c

- Vanilla extract- One teaspoon

- Kosher salt- A pinch.

Directions

Start by chilling the coconut oil in the refrigerator for about three hours. You can do it overnight.

Take out the coconut cream, and pour it in a big bowl. Leave the remaining liquid in the can.

Take out a hand mixer and beat till it is very creamy. Allow it rest.

Take out a big bowl, and use a mixer to beat the heavy cream till you notice that soft peaks have formed. You can then whisk in the vanilla and sweetener.

Whisk the whipped coconut to the whipped cream, then toss them in the loaf pan.

Allow them to freeze for close to five hours.

Sugar-free cheesecake

What You Need

- Almond flour- Half c

- Coconut flour- Half c

- Shredded coconut- Quarter c

- Melted butter- Half c

- Cream cheese- Three. Eight ounces

- Sour cream- Sixteen ounces

- Stevia- One tablespoon

- Pure vanilla extract- Two teaspoons

- Eggs- Three

- Strawberries- Sliced.

Directions

Start by preheating the oven to 200.

Start to make the crust:

Take out your spring form pan, and grease it, before covering the edges and bottoms with foil.

Take out a medium bowl, and toss in the butter, coconut and flours. Put the crust into the pan's bottom, and let it move to the sides of the pan.

Leave the pan in the refrigerator for a period. Use this time to have the filling made.

Have the filling made:

Take out a big bowl, and toss in the sour cream and cream cheese. Beat them, then whisk in the vanilla and stevia.

Toss in the eggs, and mix them. Ensure that the filling is spread well on the crust.

Leave the cheesecake in the pan, and put it in the middle rack of the oven.

Be careful as you pour boiling water in the pan till it reaches halfway.

Allow it bake for about one hour, till you notice that it jiggles lightly in the middle. Switch off the oven, but let the cake sit in the oven. Keep the door open a bit for one hour.

Take out the pan from its water bath, and remove the foil.

Leave it in the refrigerator for about five hours.

You can throw in some strawberries as garnish.

Chapter Eight

Frequently Asked Questions

Keto Adaptation- What Is It, And How Does It Feel Like?

What keto-adaption means is that your body has moved from using glucose as an energy source to using ketones.

It usually takes a few weeks after you start your keto diet before you notice this. This is if you flow it religiously. At first, you may see some symptoms that come with carbohydrate withdrawal, but all that change when you get used to it.

Keto flu: What is it? Is it avoidable?

The body normally needs glucose for its energy source. When the body realizes that you have cut carbs, it ma freak out, and this can be shown in keto flu. Some persons may not notice it, and others may. You may start to notice some flu symptoms, but it is for a very short while. Drink enough water, and you will be alright.

How long does it take to become keto-adapted or in a state of ketosis?

Research has shown that it takes a few weeks, and it can reach four weeks.

If you can cut out carbs, you can reach there quicker. If you want to speed the process, you can also exercise. Exercise will force the body to use its stored up fat.

What does ketosis mean?

When you are in the state of ketosis, your liver is creating a large number of ketones, which the body, especially the brain uses as an energy source or fuel. To work out well, you need to reduce your carbs drastically, while consuming a high amount of fats, and moderate protein.

How can I tell if I am in ketosis?

It is quite easy to tell, though you can use a breathalyzer to test it or carry out a urine or blood test to know for sure.

If you are in a state of ketosis, you will notice that your mouth is now metallic and fruity. This is what is known as keto breath. This shows that your body is running on ketones.

You will realize that you have become a lot more alert and sharp.

What may make me lose the state of ketosis, and how can I get back into it quickly?

It is hard to get into the state of ketosis, but a lot easier. The moment you eat a food that is high in carbs, your body will no longer be in a state of ketosis. The human body is wired to use glucose as an energy source. Immediately it sees carbs; it makes use of it. You can get back to ketosis by doing the same thing that got you there in the first place.

Do I need to incorporate carbohydrate re-feed days?

There are varying kinds of keto diets, and some offer you the necessary flexibility to add carb re-feed days.

These are great for those that are just starting keto diet, those that are active and need carbs for their workout, and those that had no choice but to eat carbs once in a while because of their social environment.

What is the difference between a low-carbohydrate diet and a ketogenic diet?

Don't confuse low carb foods and ketogenic diets. Consuming foods that contain close 150 grams of carbs daily can be said to be low carbs, but ketogenic needs something else.

To be in ketosis, you need to consume carbs of below 50g. Keto diet is moderate in protein and high in fat.

Conclusion

On your journey to eating healthily or shedding weight, one thing is sure; Ketogenic lifestyle can help. Gone are those days when you had to spend all your money drinking one pill or the other and pumping yourself with harmful substances all in the name of trying to lose weight. Ketogenic lifestyle can offer you this without you spending a lot of money. What else are you awaiting? Eat healthily and shed weight, without sacrificing good taste.

The complete Keto Diet

2019

21-day meal plan step by step

Keto Diet Meal, breakfast, lunch, dinner and dessert

By

J.S. JOZEF

Volume 2

Introduction

When we hear the word, 'keto', our minds usually dwell on weight loss. Keto is far more than that. The creators of the diet had the mind of using it to treat epilepsy, and it worked effortlessly well. Once better anticonvulsant medications came on board, its usage reduced. Over the years, it was noticed that keto could do more than treat epilepsy, it can help in the treatment of Alzheimer's disease and even shed weight.

A lot of persons have embraced the diet as one that allows them to remain fit, and lose weight without stress, though some sacrifices have to be made. You have to wat healthily. One thing that makes the keto diet stand out from the rest is that you don't have to sacrifice your need for sweet things and eat only bland foods.

You will have to toss those sweets that are high in carbs and sugar, but you can embrace keto sweets and snacks that are delicious and sugar-free. Who said your craving couldn't be cured in a ketogenic lifestyle?

Chapter One

Understanding what the Ketogenic diet is

The ketogenic diet is a diet that has a high amount of fats, moderate amount of protein and low amounts of carbs. All three features have to be there. Eating low carbs foods while eating foods high in protein can't be described as keto. This is because eating foods that are high in protein are similar to eating high carbs foods. When the body has excess protein, it turns it to glucose. The fats have to be high; the protein has to be moderate, while the carbs have to be low.

Ketogenic diet started when researchers in the early 1920s wanted to mimic the same effects that fasting had on epilepsy. It was noticed then that when a person fasted, the seizure he had reduced. Scientists wanted to do the same thing without people going without foods. It was noticed that the effects were replicated. Those kids that had epilepsy noticed that their seizures reduced, even after they stopped taking the diet. When good anticonvulsant medications came out, the need for a keto diet to treat epilepsy reduced.

In the case of weight loss, it is noticed that fasting can get us to the state of ketosis. This is the main reason we do a ketogenic diet. We want to be in the state of ketosis. At this state, the body turns the stored up fats to ketones, and use it as an energy source. When someone fasts, the person tends to use up stored up fats, but it is unhealthy. It is advisable to avoid fasting and opt for a safer means of getting into the state of ketosis, through a ketogenic diet.

Your body is given the nutrients it needs to survive while you lose weight. This is a classic case of killing two birds with a stone.

Chapter Two

Are You On A Ketogenic Diet?

It is common to hear a lot of persons complain that they don't know if they are in the state of ketosis. While on the journey to losing weight through a ketogenic diet, one thing is sure you can easily tell if you have reached the state of ketosis. Bellows are ways to tell:

1. Increased ketones

If you want to be sure if you are in a state of ketosis, you can draw a blood sample and take it for a test. The blood sample will tell how high your ketone levels are.

When you have a high amount of ketones in your body, you are in a state of ketosis. A breathalyzer can also pick up from your breath if you are in a state of ketosis. You can get the doctor to run a test on your urine to see your level of ketosis. Urine and breath tests aren't as reliable as the blood test.

If you don't want to test it in the hospital, you can get a home testing kit that can show you the levels of blood ketones. If you are in the nutritional ketosis, you should have ketones of about 0.5–3 millimoles per liter.

You can opt for indicator strips to see the levels of the urine. Buy your ketone testing kits online, and run the test at home.

2. Weight loss

This is one symptom that you will notice. You don't need any test kit to tell you that you have lost weight. When you are in ketosis, you should notice your body shedding weight.

This is because your body no longer has access to a high amount of carbs. Hence it has to use the stored up fats as energy. It first turns the stored up fats to ketones.

If you are in a state of ketosis, you should be losing weight.

3. Thirst

When you are in a state of ketosis, you start to notice that you are very thirsty. This is usually because you are losing water. When you are in a state of ketosis, you urinate a lot and need water. Hence you are a lot thirsty.

When you have a high amount of ketones in your body, you will notice that you are shedding a lot of water and electrolytes.

It is advisable that you drink a lot of water and liquids while on a keto diet. You need to balance the water that you are constantly losing.

4. Muscle cramps and spasms

When you are dehydrated a lot of suffering from the electrolyte imbalances, you will notice that your muscles are suffering from cramps. The electrolytes that you lose during keto are those things that transport the electrical signals from one cell to the other.

When these substances are low, you will notice that the electrical messages aren't passing well, and this could lead to spasms and muscle contractions.

It is advisable to drink a lot of water and liquids to avoid the symptoms of imbalance.

5. Headaches

When you are in a state of ketosis, you will notice that you have headaches. This isn't the case of every one. Why does this happen? Usually, this headache lasts for a day but less than a week.

The headaches are caused because your body is trying to adapt to the keto diet. Since you are consuming little carbs, the body has to adapt to the new energy source, ketones.

It could also be caused by electrolyte imbalances and dehydration. Whatever you do, consume a lot of water and liquids.

If you notice that your headache passes three days, see your doctor immediately, as it happens only at the initial stage of keto.

6. Fatigue and weakness

When a person is starting a ketogenic diet, there is a tendency of the person feeling weak. This occurs because the body is adapting to burning ketones instead of glucose. Glucose usually gives a quick burst of energy, unlike ketones. In a few days, the tiredness disappears because your body adapts to ketones. After a while on the keto diet, your energy level will increase, and you may need even more energy than someone that's not on the keto diet.

If you don't notice your energy coming back in a few weeks, you should consider talking to your physician.

7. Stomach complaints

When you make changes to your diet, your body starts to act up. That's the basic truth. This is why you start having stomach upsets when you travel out to a strange land and dine on exotic cuisines. You will realize that you have tummy complaints. Your body is not yet used to the food, but after a while, the stomach complaints stop because your body has adjusted. The same can be said for the ketogenic lifestyle.

You may notice some stomach complaints, but it is for a short while.

To help solve this, you should consider taking a lot of fluids and water. Try and eat foods that are rich in fiber, as well as non-starchy vegetables. This helps to reduce constipation.

8. Changes in sleep

When you start your ketogenic lifestyle initially, you may notice some changes to your sleeping habits. Before you know it, you are waking up at night, or having problems sleeping. This is because your body is getting used to the new diet. Once all that change, you start to sleep well

9. Bad breath

One consequence of ketosis is ketosis breath. You may notice that you have metallic breath. This happens as a result of the ketones being ejected from your body through both your urine and breath. At times, you may see your breath metallic. Other times, it may be fruity.

You can brush your teeth multiple times in a day and use sugar-free gums. They can help. After a while, your breath returns to normal.

10. Better focus and concentration

Do you know that studies show that those who are subscribers to ketogenic lifestyle have better concentration and focus? Yes, you read that right.

At first, when you start the keto diet, you may notice headaches and tiredness. This is for short while as the body adapts to the diet. After a while, you no longer see the symptoms.

If you use a keto diet for a while and religiously follow, you will notice that your clarity level has improved. Before you know it, you become a lot of focus. A study on epileptic patient showed that those who took up the keto diet become alert and attentive. Before you know it, they didn't have to battle with alert issues.

It was noticed that their level of alertness in the cognitive tests they did improve.

Chapter Three

How Does It Work

A lot of persons use a ketogenic diet for one reason or the other. It could be to shed weight or to treat epilepsy or Alzheimer's disease. Whatever the case may be, you will face the same thing when you take a keto diet.

Immediately you cut down on your consumption of carbs; you tend to notice that the amount of carbs in your food has reduced.

Before you cut the carb, the body usually burnt glucose, a product of the carbs. When you take in the carb, it is digested into glucose and used as an energy source. The glucose is transported by the blood around the body, especially the brain and the cells. The brain uses up glucose as an energy source to function well. Since you are eating a lot of foods that are high in carbs, the body continues to store up fats. Before you know it, you are increasing in weight and size.

When you have had enough and decided to lose weight, you can try out the keto diet and combine it with exercise, though not compulsory. A lot of persons use both to force their bodies into a state of ketosis quickly and burn off the burnt fat.

When you embrace keto, you toss away those foods that are high in carbs and embrace those that are high in fats.

Whatever you do while on a keto diet, your foods should be high in fats, moderate in protein and low in carbs. Do not eat foods that are high in carbs because it could ruin your efforts. The body loves glucose, and immediately it sights high amount of carbs, even when it is in a state of ketosis, it throws the state of ketosis one side and embraces the glucose once more. When you eat foods that are high in protein, it is bad, as the body can transform excess protein to glucose.

What Happens When You Take Keto Friendly Diet

At first, when you consume a keto diet, you may notice keto flu. What is that? It is common to see a lot of those who are new to the ketogenic lifestyle feel some flu-like symptoms. Why does this happen?

When you take foods high in fats, and low in carbs, the body tries to adapt to the change. This means that the body won't have access to glucose any longer. The brain will try to adapt to its new energy source, ketones, and this can lead to headaches and nausea.

It could be as a result of you using the loo a lot. When a person is new to keto, he or she tends to urinate a lot. Why? It is simple. The person is losing a lot of electrolytes and water, hence needs replacement. You take a lot of water, as it can help.

Once you start reducing the number of carbs you take, the body, especially the liver takes the fats consumed and turn them to ketones and fatty acid. The ketones are the energy source, and they take the place of glucose. They are used by the body to carry out their daily activities. That's not all, as the body starts to use the stored up fats. You see all those stored up fats that once remained untouched; the body starts to convert them to ketones. Before you know it, you are shedding weight effortlessly. At this stage, you are in ketosis. To prevent yourself from falling out of this state, you need to keep eating what you are eating.

hapter Four

Top 10 Foods You Need to Avoid

While you decide to embrace the ketogenic diet for one reason or the other, whether to shed weight or not, it is important to note that you should avoid some unhealthy foods. The one that tops the list are foods high in carbs. As much as we want you to eat foods that are high in carbs, we advise that you avoid those that have unhealthy fats like margarine. Whatever food high in fat that you cook must be healthy fats.

To prevent your body from falling out of the prided ketosis that took you weeks to get into, there are some foods that you should consider avoiding, and they are:

1. High-carb sauces

You see those sauces that you used while eating high carbs foods; they should be avoided. When you walk into the grocery store to buy a sauce, it is important to check it is keto friendly and without sugar. Some sauces that you should be cautious about are sweet salad dressing, barbecue sauce, as well as dipping sauces.

2. Bread and baked products

It is important to clamp down on the number of baked products that you consume. Many of them are high in carbs like a doughnut, rolls, white bread, cookies, crackers and so on. If you must eat baked products, ensure that they are made from keto friendly ingredients.

3. Pasta

When you jump onto the keto train, you will have to do away with noodles and spaghetti. Those foods are packing a lot of carbs. If you calculate the carbs that they have, you will be scared. If you are sure about losing weight, drop them.

4. Sweets.

There is hardly a soul on earth that doesn't fancy sweets. They are appealing to the taste buds and make us happy. We all know that, but they are high in carbs. While losing weight, they need to be tossed aside. Avoid things like maple syrup, candy, coconut sugar, and agave syrup. Your body will thank you to that.

5. Grain products

Try and toss the grain aside. A lot of these cereals that you consume in the morning are so high in carbs that if consumed can ruin your keto journey. You should think of tossing your oats, rice, and wheat aside. Kiss goodbye to tortillas and you will be happy for it.

6. Sweetened beverages.

Sweet! We love sweet things. We love our soda, sports drinks, sweetened teas, and juice. A lot of us can't do without them, but they are dangerous to health.

7. Starchy vegetables.

Veggies are good, but starchy veggies should be avoided while working on losing your weight. They trump whatever progress that you have made with your keto diet. You should think of tossing foods like pumpkin, peas, corn, and potatoes aside.

Eat veggies that are low in carbs and your weight loss will surprise you.

8. Beans and legumes.

You can increase the rate of your body burning fat by trying to avoid foods that are very high in protein. You want foods that are moderate in protein. Why? You may ask. When the body doesn't see carbs, and it sees a high amount of protein, it turns that amount to glucose.

Avoid foods like kidney beans, lentils, chickpeas, and black beans.

9. Alcoholic beverages.

Alcoholic beverages and keto do not go in the same sentence except when they negate each other. The truth remains that alcoholic beverages have a high amount of carbs. If you want to save yourself the stress, you should consider avoiding them.

10. Fruit.

While on your journey to losing weight, we advise that you take fruits, but we also advise that you avoid some fruits because of their carb level. Check the carb level of fruit before you take it. Some fruits to avoid are pineapple, bananas, grapes, and citrus.

Chapter Five

Errors to avoid

The journey to losing weight can be a simple one if you understand what to do and what time. It is common to see a lot of persons wallowing in one problem or the other because they made an error. Getting into a state of ketosis is not a day's journey, and when you leave that state because of an error on your part, getting into it becomes a problem. It is advisable to know these errors and try to avoid them. The results will surprise you.

Eating enough fat.

As much as you know the keto diet has low carb content, it is important to complement it with high fat content. About seventy percent of what you consume should be healthy fats, while five percent should be carbs, and the remaining twenty percent should be protein.

When you eat fat, you will realize that you will be satisfied. Hence your carb cravings reduce. This allows you to remain in the state of ketosis.

Eating too much protein.

A lot of persons feel that once they reduce carbs, and consume a high amount of fats that they can eat a lot of protein. This is one error that should be avoided.

When you eat an excess amount of protein, one thing is sure; it is transformed into glucose using the process of gluconeogenesis.

This means that you are indirectly eating carbs. As much as you should eat a low carb diet, the protein content should be low too. We are not excluding carbs from the diet; we are just restricting it to the amount that some body parts like blood cells need to survive. If you eat a lot of protein, you have merely given the body excess protein that it could turn to glucose.

Eating hidden carbs without realizing it.

One thing that should be noted is that some foods have carbs that you do not know of. It is common to see some condiments possessing hidden carbs.

Before you buy any food, look at its label, and try to see if there is any hidden sugar. It won't take a long time to check. This can determine if you succeed or fail in your keto journey.

Not sleeping enough.

Once you have decided to get enough sleep, you are getting closer to shedding weight. Do you know that a lot of persons feel that starving themselves of sleep improve their chances of shedding weight? This is a pure fallacy. When you don't sleep, your body becomes stressed, which reduces the level of metabolism.

Before you know it, you are storing up a lot of fats. When you are fatigued because you didn't sleep, you will notice that you will want to take latte to get a boost of energy. You may also want to dine in a late snack.

It is advisable to try and get about eight hours of sleep every night, as it helps to burn fats.

Eating too many keto sweets.

A lot of persons feel that eating a lot of keto brownies, and cookies are great because they are keto friendly, and have low carbs. You see them stuffing themselves with a lot of them. Can we burst your bubbles? The fact that they have low carbs doesn't mean that you should eat a lot of them. When you eat a lot of keto sweets with low carbs, you end up eating a lot of calories. That's not all, as you created for those sweet things before you know it, you are munching on sweets high in carbs.

You should eat keto sweets once in a while.

Snacking too much.

There are currently awesome snacks that you can eat while on a ketogenic diet like nuts, avocado, and cheese. This doesn't mean that you should eat them every time because at the end, you may add a lot of calories to your body, and you will realize that you aren't losing weight.

You should eat snacks only when you notice that you are very hungry in between meals. Apart from that, stay away from them.

Not replenishing your electrolytes.

When some persons begin the keto diet, they start to feel sick, having flu symptoms. The reasons this occurs are:

When the body is no longer using glucose as its energy source, and now has to use fat, the brain has to adapt to it. This may lead to headaches and nausea.

You may be dehydrated because you will urinate a lot while on keto. If you don't drink water, this can bring a lot of issues.

If you notice the keto flu, don't be scared. This shows that your body is adapting to the keto diet. What you should do to reduce the keto flu is to take a lot of water. You need to have your electrolytes supplemented

One supplement that you should consider taking to put you in the right state is KetoLogic

BHB. It helps to treat the keto flu and ushers you quickly into ketosis.

Eating too much dairy.

A lot of persons tend to have an inflammatory response when they consume a lot of dairy products. This can affect their progress to weight loss. That's not all, like we earlier said, taking a lot of protein can inhibit weight loss.

A lot of dairy foods have both protein and fats. Some even have carbs but in a limited amount.

When you consume dairy foods, ensure that its fat content is higher than its protein and carbs content.

Eating too many calories.

A lot of persons think that one can consume as much as they want, as long as the food is keto friendly. This is misleading and should be avoided at all costs.

You should consume healthy fats in large quantity, but you should never eat more calories that can be burnt. If you eat excess food, the additional calories end up as body fat.

Usually, a normal person needs close to two thousand calories daily, but this number is dependent on some factors like activity, height, and gender.

Not drinking enough water.

Our basic health science class taught us that water is key to our health. If you fall under those that hate taking water, then there is a big problem because your rate of metabolism will drop.

You should try and take about sixty-four ounces of water daily. This helps to remove the toxins. While you start your keto journey, you need to drink a lot of water, as it helps to combat the keto flu and so on.

Chapter Six

The best ten foods you need

While on keto, some foods should be eaten, and there are some that should be avoided. Below are ten foods that you should consider eating while on a keto diet:

Nuts and Seeds

Have you tried the sunflower seeds, pumpkin seeds, macadamia nuts, almonds, and pecans? They are all awesome ways that one can get healthy fats.

They are high in fiber and without a high amount of carbs. They are easy to afford, and you can easily track your carbs with them.

You can use them as snacks or even add them to the ingredients of smoothies.

Olives

Have you tried black and green olives? They are high in healthy fats, and great for the heart. Since you are in keto, you need foods that are high in fats and low in carbs. Olives can offer you this. You can easily have them warmed up with the marinara, or even garnish zoodles with it.

Condiments

A lot of things that you will find in the condiments aisles are keto friendly, though you have to read their labels first to be sure. Some options that you consider looking at are:

- Mayo
- Ketchup
- Buffalo sauce
- Salad dressing
- Mustard.

Oils

Whatever oil you decide to buy, it is important to check if they are made up of fat. As much as keto preaches eating foods that are high in fats, they also want you to consume those that are high in healthy fats.

Some of the oils that you can consider using are:

- Coconut oil

- MCT oil

- Cooking oil- Don't forget to look at the label.

- Noncooking oil- Don't forget to look at the label.

Ghee

Yes, you read that right! Clarified butter or ghee is great for keto. You can use the shrimp, asparagus, and butter to give that saltiness that you wish for.

A lot of persons are in love with ghee, as it gives off the nuttiness unseen in usual butter. It is great to the taste buds.

Salt

You need salt. Everyone that undergoes ketogenic lifestyle needs salt. Why is this so? When your body starts to burn fat, you may tend to feel the electrolyte swings.

Before you know it, you can't stop urinating constantly. What this means is that your body is shedding a lot of electrolytes and sodium.

Taking salt helps to replace it.

Prepared Snacks

Who said you couldn't have snacks while on Keto? No one. What you can't have are processed or unhealthy snacks. Do you feel like snacking? You can munch on snacks that aren't high in carbs like

- Cheese crisps
- Pork rinds
- Pill nuts
- Meat snacks.

Flours and Thickeners

You can use keto friendly flour to bake. You don't have to stop baking just because you are on a keto diet. You can try the almond meal, almond flour, as well as coconut flour. They have a low carb, but high in fiber.

Since they come with a nutty flavor, they are great for waffles, muffins, pancakes or even cookies.

Nut Butter

A lot of traditional peanut butter comes with sugar. There is the unsweetened option that can be consumed by keto eaters. You will enjoy peanut butter without pumping yourself with lots of sugar.

You can also have access to the unsweetened almond butter. You can also make your own. Add vanilla or cinnamon to it, and you will enjoy it

Keto-approved Sweeteners

When people think of healthy living, they think of bland foods. Gone are those days when you had to eat tasteless things all in the name of following the keto lifestyle. If you love the thought of consuming pancakes, you can try it out with keto friendly sweeteners like Swerve, Splenda, Stevia and so on.

Chapter Seven

Keto-friendly recipes

Chorizo breakfast bake

What You Need

- Olive oil- A tbsp

- Red pepper- Half cup

- Onion- Half cup

- Chorizo sausages- Four oz

- Eggs- Two

- Pepper

- Salt

- Bacon- Two slices

Guidelines

Start by preheating the oven to a high temperature of 250. Try and grease the two ramekins.

Take out a skillet and place it on a stove with medium heat.

Whisk in your onion and peppers. Allow them to cook for about five minutes till you notice that they have been browned.

Have the veggies mixture shared among the two ramekins.

Have the chorizo chopped, then shared them between the ramekins.

Break the egg, and put it in every ramekin. Add the pepper, as well as the salt.

Have it baked for about twelve minutes till you notice that the egg is ready.

Have the bacon crumbled on the top. You can only serve it hot.

Cheesy single-serve Lasagna

What You Need

- Marinara- Three tbsp

- Zucchini- One

- Ricotta cheese- Two tbsp

- Mozzarella- Three oz

Guidelines

Take out a bowl that is microwave safe, then add a spoonful of the marinara sauce.

Take out the sauce and spread it on the zucchini slices. Use a tbsp of the ricotta on it.

Do the same with the other layers, as well as ricotta and sauce.

Use the other zucchini to cover it, then add the mozzarella.

Leave in the microwave for about four minutes till they are well heated, and the cheese has melted.

Mushroom Soup with Fried egg

What You Need

- Olive oil- One Tsp

- Mushrooms- Four

- Cauliflower- One hundred grams

- Vegetable broth- One cup

- Heavy cream- Three tbsp

- Cheese- Two tbsp

- Butter- One Tsp

- Egg- One

Guidelines

Take out your saucepan, and put it on a stove with medium heat. Have the oil heated.

Toss in the mushrooms, then allow them to cook till you notice they are soft. This should take six minutes.

Add your heavy cream, veggie broth, as well as riced cauliflower.

Toss in the pepper and salt. Whisk in your cheese.

Allow the soup simmer, till it has thickened to the extent that it is necessary. Then take it off the state be.

Try and have the egg fried in the butter to the extent that you want. It can be served with the soup.

Avocado Egg & salami sandwiches

What You Need

- Cloud buns- Four

- Eggs- Four

- Butter- One Tsp

- Tomato- One

- Mozzarella- One oz

- Avocado- One

- Pepper

- Salt

- Two oz of sliced salami

Guidelines

Take out the baking sheet, and line it.

Have the cloud buns put there, then leave it in an oven. Allow it there till they become golden brown.

Take out a big skillet, and put it on a stove with medium heat, then add the butter there.

Break the eggs and put them in the skillet, before you try to season them with pepper, as well as salt.

Allow the eggs to cook to the extent that they are ready, then put on every cloud bun.

Add the tomato slice, avocado, mozzarella, as well as salami on the buns.

Serve now.

Mozzarella Tuna Melt

What You Need

- Olive oil- One tbsp

- Onion- Half cup

- Mayo- Quarter cup

- Tuna- Eight oz

- Eggs- Two

- Mozzarella- Two oz

- Pepper

- Salt

- Onion- One

Guidelines

Have the skillet placed on a stove with medium heat. Put the oil there, then whisk in the onion. Allow it to cook for close to five minutes.

Have the tuna drained, then allow it flaked in the skillet. Continue to whisk in the rest of the ingredients.

Add your pepper and salt. Whisk them, and allow them to cook for about two minutes. The cheese should have melted.

Take out a bowl, and add the green onion. You can serve.

Three-cheese Pizza Frittata

What You Need

- Thawed Frozen Spinach- Ten oz

- Eggs- Six

- Olive oil- Two tbsp

- Italian seasoning- Half tsp

- Pepper

- Salt

- Ricotta cheese- Quarter cup

- Parmesan cheese- Quarter cup

- Mozzarella cheese- Two and a half oz

- Pepperoni- One oz

Guidelines

Have the oven preheated to a high temperature of 175. Take out the pie plate, then grease using cooking spray.

Have the spinach defrosted. Do this by leaving it in a microwave for about four minutes. This will drive out the water.

Break the egg, then add the olive oil, pepper, salt, and Italian seasoning. Whisk them well.

Add the parmesan cheese, ricotta cheese, as well as drained spinach, then whisk them till they form well.

Toss in a pie plate, the mixture that was formed. Add the pepperoni, as well as mozzarella.

Leave in the oven for about forty minutes. By this time, the egg has been set, while the cheese has been browned a bit.

You can then serve.

Bacon Breakfast Bombs

What You Need

- Bacon- Four slices

- Eggs- Two

- Butter- Quarter cup

- Mayo- Two tbsp

- Pepper

- Salt

Guidelines

Take out a large skillet and place it on a stove with medium heat. Put the bacon there till they become crisp.

Allow the bacon to rest for a while before you chop it. Keep the bacon grease somewhere else.

Take out a saucepan, and put water in it, then add salt. Allow it boil well.

Put the eggs there, then allow them to boil for about ten minutes. Place them in a water bath.

Allow the eggs to rest. You can then peel them well. Don't forget to cut them coarsely.

Have the eggs mashed, then whisk the butter, pepper, salt, and mayo.

Whisk the bacon grease that was kept somewhere, before you have the mixture covered. Allow them to chill for half an hour.

Have the egg mixture shared into the portion before you have them rolled into the balls. Don't forget to have them rolled in the crushed bacon.

Try and serve it instantly. The ones that are leftovers, store in the refrigerator.

Easy Cloud Buns

What You Need

- Eggs- Three

- Cream of tartar- One-eight tsp

- Cream cheese- Three oz.

Guidelines

Have the oven preheated to a high temperature of 200. Take out your baking sheet and line it up using parchment.

Whisk your egg whites till you notice that they are foamy, then you can add the cream of tartar. Whisk them well till you see that the egg whites are both opaque and shiny, showing soft peaks.

Take out a different bowl, and add the egg yolks and cream cheese. Whisk them well, and then add the egg white mixture.

On your baking sheet, put the batter and make quarter cup circles. Leave close to two inches between both of them.

Allow them to bake for about half an hour, till you notice that the buns are no longer soft.

You can then serve.

Gyro Salad With Avo-tzatziki

Prep Time: 10 minutes

What You Need

- Olive oil- A tbsp

- Lamb meat- One pound

- Onion- Half

- Chicken broth- Quarter cup

- Lemon juice- Four tsp

- Dried oregano- Half tsp

- Dried thyme- Half tsp

- Cucumber- Half

- Avocado- One

- Mint- Half tsp

- Dill- One Tsp

- Romaine lettuces- Six cups

Guidelines

Take out your big skillet, then put it on a stove with medium heat. Put the oil there, then the lamb.

Allow them to cook for about three minutes, and toss well. You can add your onion now.

Continue to cook well till the lamb is well cooked. Add the onion there, then whisk them well, before you add the thyme, oregano, lemon juice, and chicken broth.

Add the pepper, as well as the salt. Allow it simmer well for about five minutes.

Have the cucumber grated well, before you use a clean towel to remove the moisture of any kind.

Put the cucumber into the food processor, before you toss in the lemon juice, salt, dill, mint, as well as avocado. Continue until they become smooth.

Have them served.

Cabbage and Sausage Skillet

What You Need

- Sausage links- Six

- Cabbage- Half

- Butter- Two tbsp

- Sour cream- Quarter cup

- Mayo- Quarter cup

- Pepper

- Salt

Guidelines

Take out a skillet, and place it on a stove with medium heat. Put the sausage there till they are browned well. Remove the sausage, and slice well.

Put the skillet in the stove on medium heat again, then toss the butter into it.

Add your cabbage, then whisk till it becomes wilted. This should take over four minutes.

Whisk in the sausage that has been stirred in the wilted cabbage. Add your mayo, as well as sour cream.

Toss the pepper, as well as salt. Allow them to simmer for about ten minutes.

You can serve well.

Chicken Zoodle Alfredo

What You Need

- Chicken breasts- Six oz

- Olive oil- One tbsp

- Pepper

- Salt

- Butter- Two tbsp

- Heavy cream- Quarter cup

- Parmesan cheese- Quarter cup

- Zucchini- Two hundred grams.

Guidelines

Have the skillet placed on a stove with medium heat. Put the oil there.

Add the pepper, as well as salt to the chicken. Toss the chicken to the heated skillet.

Have them cooked for about six minutes till it is cooked. Have the chicken cut into strips.

Put the skillet on the stove on the medium heat again, then toss the butter.

Add your parmesan cheese, as well as heavy cream. Allow them to become thick.

Have the zucchini spiralized before you toss it in the mixture that has the chicken.

Continue to cook the zucchini until it becomes soft. It should take over three minutes. Try and serve it hot.

Pan-fried Pepperoni Pizzas

What You Need

- Eggs- Six

- Parmesan cheese- Six tbsp

- Psyllium husk powder- Three tbsp

- Italian seasoning- One and a half tsp

- Olive oil- Three tbsp

- Tomato sauce- Nine tbsp

- Mozzarella- Four and a half oz

- Pepperoni- One and a half oz

- Chopped basil- Three tbsp

Guidelines

Take out a blender, and toss in the parmesan, eggs, Italian seasoning, psyllium husk powder, as well as salt.

Continue to blend well till you notice that it smooth. This should take close to a minute. Allow it to rest well for about five minutes.

Take out a skillet and place it on a stove with medium heat. Add a tbsp of oil.

Have one-third of the batter added to the skillet. Allow them to spread into a circle, and then brown well.

Have the pizza crust flipped, till it becomes brown.

Take off the crust and put it in the baking sheet. Do it over and over again using the extra batter.

Add three tbsp of the tomato sauce on every crust.

Add the cheese and pepperoni. Allow them to broil till you notice that the cheese has been browned.

Add your basil. Slice before you serve.

Easy Cheeseburger Salad

What You Need

- Beef- Seven oz

- Mayo- Three tbsp

- Pepper

- Salt

- Pickles- One tbsp

- Mustard- One Tsp

- Ketchup- Half tsp

- Smoked paprika

- Romaine lettuce- Three oz

- Tomatoes- One-third cup

- Cheddar cheese- Quarter cup

Guidelines

Have the ground beef browned. You can then add the pepper and salt.

Try and remove the fat from the beef. Take it out of the heat.

Take out a blender, and add the paprika, ketchup, mustard, pickles, and mayo.

Have the mixture blended well.

Take out a bowl, and add the cheddar cheese, tomatoes, lettuce, and ground beef.

Coat dressing gently on it. You can then serve.

Pepper Jack Sausage Egg Muffins

What You Need

- Ground sausage- Ten oz

- Garlic powder- Quarter tsp

- Onion- Half cup

- Pepper

- Salt

- Eggs- Three

- Heavy cream- Two tbsp

- Pepper Jack Cheese- Half cup

Guidelines

Have the oven preheated to a high temperature of 250. Take out the three ramekins and grease them well using cooking spray.

Take out a bowl, and add the pepper, salt, garlic powder, onion, and ground sausage.

Have the sausage mix shared well using the ramekins. Have them pressed into the sides, as well as the bottom. Allow the middle to be opened.

Have the eggs whisked, then toss the pepper, salt, and heavy cream.

Have the egg mixture shared in the sausage cups, then toss the shredded chess.

Leave them in the oven for about thirty minutes till the eggs have been set. Ensure that the cheese is browned.

You can then serve.

Mozzarella Veggie-loaded Quiche

What You Need

- Almond flour- Six tbsp

- Parmesan cheese- One tbsp

- Eggs- Two

- Bacon- Two

- Frozen spinach- Quarter cup

- Zucchini- Quarter cup

- Mozzarella cheese- Quarter cup

- Tomatoes- Four

- Heavy cream- One tbsp

- Chives- One Tsp

Guidelines

Take out a bowl, and whisk in the parmesan and almond flour. Toss in the salt and egg. Whisk well till it becomes soft.

Take out a quiche pan, and ensure that the dough is pressed. Allow it to be spread evenly.

Have the sides, as well as bottom scored. Allow the dough bake for about seven minutes. It should be heated to a high temperature of 225.

Take it out and allow it cool well.

Take out a skillet, and brown the bacon with it, then place it in a quiche pan.

Have zucchini, spinach, tomatoes, and cheese sprinkled there.

Have the remaining egg whisked with chives, heavy cream, salt, and pepper. Add the mixture poured in the quiche.

Allow it to bake for about twenty-five minutes till the egg has been set.

Savory Ham And Cheese Waffles

What You Need

- Eggs- Four

- Egg White Protein Powder- Two scoops

- Baking powder- One Tsp

- Butter- One-third cup

- Salt- half tsp

- Ham- One oz

- Cheddar cheese- Quarter cup

Guidelines

Break two eggs, and beat their yolks, then add the baking powder, protein, salt, and butter using a bowl.

Add the cheddar cheese and chopped ham to the mixture.

Take out another bowl, and beat in the egg whites, as well as the salt till you notice the stiff peaks forming.

Toss in the egg whites that have been beaten to the egg yolk mixture in two different batches.

Take out your waffle maker, and preheat it before you grease it. Add a quarter batter cup before you close it.

Continue to cook till you notice that the waffle has turned a golden brown hue. This should take close to four minutes. You can remove them.

Have the waffle maker reheated, then do the same with the other batter.

Have the oil in that skillet heated; have your eggs fried with pepper and salt.

You can then serve the hot waffles. Don't forget to top it using fried egg.

Chapter Eight

Tips for losing 21 pounds in 21 days

Losing those pounds do not have to be stressful as long as you know what you are doing. With these tips, you get closer to shedding twenty-one pounds in twenty-one days. The great aspect of them is that they can easily be done.

Drink A Lot Of Water

This is something that shouldn't be ignored. You have to gulp down as much water as possible. It is really bad that a lot of persons hate drinking water. The major source of liquid to them is alcohol or soft drinks. Taking a lot of water helps the body to remove those toxins, improve on digestion, clamp down on constipation and to bloat. It even goes ahead to improve metabolism and internal PH. It is advisable to drink about four liters of water daily.

When you wake up in the morning, one of the first things you should do apart from brushing your teeth is to drink at least two glasses of water that's at room temperature. It is advisable to add fenugreek seeds to it, as they help to improve the metabolism.

You can try to create homemade detox water by tossing in mint leaves, cumin, garlic, and cucumber. This allows the body to function well.

Stop Eating Junk Food, Sugar And Processed Food

This is definitely for your good. Try and avoid junk foods of all kind for three weeks. When watching Netflix at night, don't be tempted to munch on the sugar. Don't worry, do it for three weeks without cheating, and you will be amazed by the awesome results you will notice.

Throw away every type of unhealthy food that is laced with sugar, preservatives and a large amount of sodium. What should be in your kitchen are low calories foods and whole foods.

If the craving for sugary things come, opt for yogurts that are low in calories, and top them with peaches or figs.

Try and add a piece of dark chocolate once you are done with dinner. It can help with the craving.

Eat Different Kinds of Fruits and Veggies

On your journey to shedding pounds, it is advisable to try out different kinds of veggies and fruits. I will advise you to try out three kinds of fruits, and five kinds of vegetables daily. Why is this so? When you consume veggies and fruits, you introduce a high amount of minerals, vitamins, dietary fiber, as well as phytonutrients to the body. They go a long way to improve the level of satiety while reducing the rate of absorption of those fat molecules.

Veggies and fruits have little calories and can enhance the movement of your bowel, while your body builds its immunity level. As your body cells improve in their functioning, your stored up fat is used as an energy source. Before you know it, you are losing weight.

Avoid White Carbs

When we talk of bad carbs or white carbs, we are speaking of delicacies such as sugar, flour, crackers, white rice, cereals, and pasta. When you look at these foods, one thing is sure- they are highly refined and come bearing little nutrients. Their calorie level shoots through the roof. When you munch on bad carbs, the level of your glucose level increase. Since they are digested quickly, before you know it, you are hungry again and munching on those high-calorie meals.

You should try out healthier varieties such as beans, cauliflower, turnip, and white potatoes.

Eat On Time and Reduce the amount of food you munch on

When I hear people complain that they don't eat early or starve for a long time, yet their weight seems to be increasing, I know that those methods are futile. Starving and not eating on time shouldn't be what you use when you want to shed weight.

What you should do is to eat on time and control the size of the food you consume. Do you know that the amount of food you eat adds a lot too if you gain weight or not.

One thing that you should know is that you may have a healthy eating habit, but if your body is unable to digest, absorb, as well as remove toxins quickly, your entire system may have a huge problem to deal with.

This could worsen into a slow metabolism, thereby improving the blood glucose, as well as blood pressure. Before you know it, your weight is increasing.

This is why you should try and eat breakfast, and dinner before night. Don't try eating snacks late, and ensure you rest well.

When you starve yourself, your body enters famine mode, thereby forcing the body cells to keep everything eaten into a state of fat. When the hunger comes at night, you can munch on fruits instead of snacks. Like always, don't forget to drink lots of water.

Watch How You Eat

I mean you should do it. You are probably wondering why we asked you to do this. Well, take a ride with us. It is important to note that these tips are short term ones to make you lose the necessary weight.

When you sit in front of a mirror and watch yourself eat, you stop overeating. While you eat, try and shut your mouth as you chew. This prevents you from taking in air and improves the functioning of your digestive system.

While you serve yourself, opt for a smaller plate and spoon, as they prevent you from eating a lot of food. Try and eat gradually, and eliminate all forms of distractions such as watching TV, using the phone and so on.

Work It Out

One thing that you should note is that when you lose weight quickly, you may gain the weight back, and come bearing loose skin.

To look healthy and toned, if it is advisable that you start exercising. If you don't fancy running or the gym, you should think of trying yoga. You can as well swim or even dance.

If you love the gym, you can consider trying bodyweight training, and maybe, you can flaunt that cute body you worked on at the beach.

When you work out, your metabolism increases, and you will be able to sleep well. If you want to work on your confidence, you should consider working on.

Get Your Beauty Sleep

A lot of persons feel that when they sleep a lot, they will gain weight. That's a pure fallacy, as the opposite is the case. Not sleeping well can improve your weight gain. If you don't sleep for about eight hours, your body cells won't be able to process the food properly. They won't be able to get rid of those toxins. When you rarely sleep, your healing process reduces, and you become a lot stressed.

Before you know it, you are gaining a lot of weight, and fatigued, even when you have not carried out anything throughout the day.

Chapter Nine

21-day meal plan shopping list

Are you thinking of starting a ketogenic diet, and wondering what to eat? This 21-day meal plan can help.

Day 1

For breakfast, try out the Chorizo Breakfast Bake.

For lunch, you can try out the Sesame Pork Lettuce Wraps.

For dinner, you can try out the Avocado Lime Salmon.

The total calories of the food for day 1 are 1,520. As for fat, it is 109g.

For protein, it is 110g. The net carbs of the foods are 16g.

Day 2

For breakfast, consume the leftover chorizo breakfast bake.

For lunch, try out the Thick Cut Bacon with spiced pumpkin soup leftover

For dinner, try out the Avocado Lime Salmon.

The total calories of the foods are 1,570. As for fat, it is 124g. For protein, it is 92g, and the net carbs are 16g.

Day 3

For breakfast, try out Baked Eggs in Avocado.

For lunch, try out Easy Beef Curry Rosemary.

For dinner, try out Roasted Chicken and Veggies.

The total calories are 1,700. As for fat, it is 128.5g. As for protein, it is 103g, and the net carbs are 22g.

Day 4

For breakfast, try out the Lemon Poppy Ricotta, pancakes and three slices of bacon.

For lunch, try out the pumpkin soup, avocado.

For dinner, try out the roasted chicken and veggies that were left over.

The total calories of the day's foods are 1,665. As for fat, it is 130g. For protein, it is 95.5g, and the net carbs for the day are 23.5g.

Day 5

For breakfast, try out the lemon poppy ricotta pancakes, as well as the thick cut bacon.

For lunch, try out the porridge and bacon.

For dinner, try out the leftover beef curry, as well as cheesy sausage and mushroom skillet.

The total calories of the foods are 1,670. For fat, it is 112g, protein is 100g, and net carbs are 33.5g.

Day 6

For breakfast, try out the sweet blueberry coconut porridge that was left over.

For lunch, try out the Easy beef curry.

For dinner, try out the lamb chops and garlic, and Rosemary.

The total calories of the foods are 1,625. For fat, it is 108g; protein is 110.5g.

Shopping List For The First Week

For the Protein, you should consider shopping for the following:

Seventeen slices of bacon

A pound of the beef

Four chicken thighs, deskinned and boneless.

Four oz of Chorizo sausages

Seven eggs

Two lamb chops

Six oz pork

Six oz Italian sausage

DAIRY

A cup of almond milk

A pound of butter

Two tbsps of cheddar cheese

Five tbsps of heavy creams

Half cup of mozzarella cheese

Six oz of ricotta cheese

PRODUCE

A quarter pound of asparagus

Two avocados

Small green bell pepper

Medium red bell pepper

Sixty grams of blueberries

Four leaves of butter lettuce

Two carrots

One stalk of celery

A bunch of cilantro

One head of garlic

One piece of ginger

One lemon

One lime

Four oz mushrooms

Two onion

One parsnip

One rosemary

One zucchini

FOR PANTRY ITEMS

- A quarter cup of almond flour

- Balsamic vinegar

- Baking powder

- One cup of chicken broth

- A quarter cup of coconut flour

- One coconut milk can

- Curry powder

- Coconut oil

- Dried thyme

- Dried oregano

- Garlic powder

- Egg white protein powder

- Liquid Stevia

- Olive oil

- A quarter cup of marinara sauce

- Pepper

- Onion powder

- Half cup of Pumpkin puree

- One tbsp of Poppy seeds

- Salt

- Powdered erythritol

- One tbsp of sesame seeds

- Sesame oil

- A quarter cup of shaved coconut

Day 7

For breakfast, try out the far busting vanilla protein smoothy

For lunch, try out the cheeseburger salad.

For dinner, try out the chicken zoodle Alfredo.

The total calories of the foods are 1,530. For fat,

it is 113.5g, protein is 107.5g, and the net carbs are 18.5g.

Day 8

For breakfast, try out the ham and cheese.

For lunch, try out the waffles and bacon.

For dinner, try out the pepperoni pizzas cabbage, as well as sausage skillet.

The total calories of the foods are 1,670.

For fat, it is 129g, protein is 103g, and the net carbs are 20.5g.

Day 9

For breakfast, try out the three cloud buns and three tablespoons of peanut butter, as well as bacon.

For lunch, try out the Three-Cheese

Pizza Frittata and bacon.

For dinner, try out the pepperoni, ham, as well as bacon.

For lunch, try out the Three-Cheese

Pizza Frittata and bacon.

For dinner, try out the pepperoni, ham, as well as Cheddar Stromboli.

The total calories of the foods are 1,640.

For fat, it is 130.5g, protein is 100.5g, and the net carbs are 20.5g.

Day 10

For breakfast, try out the mozzarella veggie loaded.

For lunch, try out the quiche, bacon, cheeseburger salad.

For dinner, try out the gyro salad and

Avo-tzatziki. The total calories of the foods are 1,580. For fat, it is 104.5g, protein is 117.5g, and the net carbs are 33g.

Day 11

For breakfast, try out the Pepper Jack Sausage, egg muffins and bacon.

For lunch, try out the pepperoni pizza.

For dinner, try out the cabbage and sausage skillet that was left over.

The total calories are 1,650. For fat, it is 127.5g, protein is 101g, and the net carbs are 29g.

Day 12

For breakfast, try out the ham and cheese waffles, and bacon.

For lunch, try out the cabbage and sausage skillet.

For dinner, try out the chicken zoodle Alfredo. The total calories of the foods are 1,620. For fat, it is 119g, protein is 119g, and the net carbs are 18.5g.

Day 13

For breakfast, try out pepper jack sausage egg muffins and bacon.

For lunch, try out the pepperoni pizza that is left over.

For dinner, try out the gyro salad and Avo-Tzatziki that are left over.

The total calories of the foods are 1,595. For fat, it is 116g, protein is 110g, and the net carbs are 15.5g.

Day 14

For breakfast, try out the pepper jack sausage egg muffins and half avocado.

For lunch, try out the cabbage, sausage skills, and bacon.

For dinner, try out the gyro salad and Avo-Tzatziki.

The total calories of the foods are 1,605. For fat, it is 102g, protein is 102g, and net carbs are 22.5g.

Shopping List

PROTEIN

You need the following to make your second-week meals:

- Eleven Bacon

- Seven oz beef

- Ten ounces sausage

- Six oz chicken breast

- Fifteen eggs

- One oz ham

- One pound lamb

- One and a half oz pepperoni

- Six sausage links

DAIRY

- For dairy, try the following:

- A quarter cup of almond milk

- A three-quarter cup of butter

- Half cup of cheddar cheese

- One cup of heavy cream

- Half cup of mayo

- One and a half cups of mozzarella cheese

- Three-quarter of parmesan cheese

- Half cup of pepper jack cheese

- A quarter cup of sour cream

- A quarter cup of whipped cream

PRODUCE

- Two avocados

- One Basil

- Half head of cabbage

- One chive

- One cucumber

- One dill

- One lemon

- One mint

- One onion

- Seven and half cups of romaine lettuce

- Quarter cup of frozen spinach

- Four tomatoes

- One-third of tomatoes

- Two cups of zucchini

PANTRY ITEMS

- Six tbsp of almond flour

- Quarter cup of chicken broth

- Baking powder

- Dried thyme

- Dried oregano

- Coconut oil

- Three scoops of vanilla

- Egg white protein powder,

- Italian season

- Garlic powder

- Olive oil

- Mustard

- Ketchup

- Black pepper

- Smoked paprika

- Salt

- Erythritol

- Psyllium husk powder

- Low car tomato sauce, and

- Vanilla extract

Day 15

For breakfast, try out the three tablespoons of peanut butter, three cloud buns, as well as bacon.

For lunch, try out the mozzarella tuna.

For dinner, try out the cheesy single serve lasagna.

The total calories are 1,605. For fat, it is 116.5g. For protein, it is 114.5g, and their net carbs are 28.5g.

Day 16

For breakfast, try out the Bacon Breakfast Bombs Avocado.

For lunch, try out the Egg & Salami Sandwiches.

For dinner, try out the Crispy Chipotle Chicken Thighs.

The total calories are 1,525. For fat, it is 118.5g, protein is 99.5g, and the net carbs are 12g.

Day 17

For breakfast, try out the Three-Cheese Pizza Frittata and Bacon.

For lunch, try out the mozzarella tuna melt.

For dinner, try out the Pepperoni, Ham, as well as Cheddar Stromboli.

The total calories are 1,660. For fat, it is 121g, protein is 119g, and net carbs are 22.5g.

Day 18

For breakfast, try out the three cloud buns and three tablespoons of peanut butter, as well as bacon.

For lunch, try out the Three-Cheese

Pizza Frittata and bacon.

For dinner, try out the pepperoni, ham, as well as bacon.

For lunch, try out the Three-Cheese

Pizza Frittata and bacon.

For dinner, try out the pepperoni, ham, as well as Cheddar Stromboli.

The total calories of the foods are 1,640.

For fat, it is 130.5g, protein is 100.5g, and the net carbs are 20.5g.

Day 19

For breakfast, try out the bacon breakfast bombs.

For lunch, try out the Avocado, Egg &

Salami Sandwiches, as well as bacon.

For dinner, try out the Crispy Chipotle

Chicken Thighs.

The total calories are 1,625. For fat, it is 126.5g, protein is 106.5g, and the net carbs are 12.5g.

Day 20

For breakfast, try out the Three-Cheese Pizza Frittata, and bacon.

For lunch, try out the Pepperoni, Ham,

and Cheddar Stromboli.

For dinner, try out the Spring Salad with Steak and Sweet Dressing.

The total calories are 1,585.

For fat, it is 120.5g, protein is 108g, and the net carbs are 13.5g.

Day 21

For breakfast, try out the Three-Cheese Pizza Frittata and Bacon.

For lunch, try out the Mushroom Soup, as well as Fried Egg and bacon.

For dinner, try out the Spring Salad, Steak and Sweet Dressing are leftover.

The total calories are 1,665. For fat, it is 130.5g, protein is 110g, and the net carbs are 13.5g.

Shopping List

PROTEIN

- Twenty three bacon
- Seven oz of beef
- Twelve oz of chicken thighs
- Nineteen eggs
- Six oz of ham

- Three oz of pepperoni

- Two oz of salami

- Eight oz of tuna

DAIRY

- Seven tbsps of butter

- Two tbsps of shredded cheddar cheese

- Four oz of sliced cheddar cheese

- Three oz of cream cheese

- Three tbsp of heavy cream

- Six tbsp of mayo

- One oz of mozzarella

- Three and quarter mozzarella

- A quarter cup of parmesan cheese

- One-third of ricotta cheese.

PRODUCE

- One avocado

- One hundred grams of cauliflower

- One garlic

- Four mushrooms

- One green onion

- One onion

- Four raspberries

- Ten cups of salad greens

- Three cups of fresh spinach

- One frozen spinach

- One tomato

- One zucchini

PANTRY ITEMS

- A quarter cup of almond flour
- Chipotle Chili
- Baking powder
- Three tbsp of coconut flour
- Italian season
- Cream of tartar
- Almond flour
- Three tbsp marinara
- Liquid Stevia
- Ground coriander
- Garlic powder
- Onion powder
- Olive oil
- One oz of pine nuts

- Black pepper

- Salt

- Erythritol

- Paprika- Smoked

- One cup of vegetable broth, and

- White wine vinegar.

The recipes are in chapter 7.

Conclusion

When we are trying to lose weight, we become desperate to the extent that we are ready to swallow a lot of things. It is common to see some persons pumping themselves with pills, and at the end, they are left with one health issue or the other. What of those that try one product or the other that claims to work magic, and the end, money is gone, and the state has worsened. Are you tired of being duped? It is time you embraced the natural process and watch what you eat. The ketogenic diet can help you lose weight without you exercising, but if you want to speed it up, you can exercise.

Ingredients for keto foods are easy to stress, and the recipes are easy to make. You don't have to stress yourself any longer, all in the name of losing weight. The awesome part of all these is that keto friendly diets are tasteful to the taste buds. You don't have to sacrifice your love for sweet things on the altar of eating healthily.